# GAPS Diet

## One Pot Delights Cookbook

Delicious Slow Cooker, Stockpot,
Skillet & Roasting Pan Recipes

# TABLE OF CONTENTS

# Bonus: Heal Your Gut Mini-Series

I am both delighted and humbled that you have chosen my book to start or continue on your gut healing journey. Eating healthily and following a specific health diet is not easy and I want to help with this as much as possible, which is why I am pleased to offer you three mini e-books from my "Heal Your Gut" mini-series, completely free of charge.

These three mini e-books will show you how to make gut healing stews and soups, as well as gut friendly breads and healthy, clean desserts.

Simply click on the link below and fill out your email address so I can send you your free mini e-books.

www.andreparker.co/freebonus

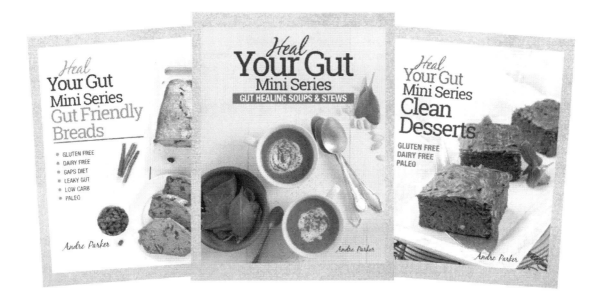

# Thank You

I want to thank you for purchasing this book and I really hope it helps you keep to your health goals. The GAPS diet completely turned my life around and I am now healthy and fit thanks to this diet. I have been compelled to write this book by my desire to help others benefit from the GAPS diet in the life-changing way that it has helped me. I hope that these easy but delicious recipes will inspire you to start or continue with the GAPS diet and put you on the road to a healthier, more active and more fulfilling life.

I would love to hear about your story and how the GAPS diet has helped you or a loved one so please feel free to email me at the address below.

If you enjoyed this book or have any suggestions, then I'd appreciate it if you would leave a review or simply e-mail me your feedback.

You can leave a review on Amazon at the link below:

www.andreparker.co/onepotreview

Or email me at:
info@andreparker.co

Warmest Regards,
Andre

# My Digestive Healing Journey

My digestive healing story started over 6 years ago. I suffered from numerous gut health issues and I had a number of different symptoms to which, I am sure, many of you reading this could relate. Some of these symptoms included constipation, chronic fatigue, weight gain, sugar addiction and carbohydrate addiction. I even had to deal with two different parasites. On top of all this, I also suffered from bacteria imbalances and overgrowth, gastritis, Helicobacter Pylori and ulcerative colitis. Due to all of the damage that had occurred in my digestive system, I also had a leaky gut. My digestive health was almost nonexistent.

I finally became fed up and decided to take responsibility for my own health. I realized that I had the power to make the choice to take charge of my own health.

Through my journey, I learned that we all have a choice to eat to feed disease or to eat to prevent, heal and radiate health. Healthy, organic and wholesome food truly is medicine.

My digestive healing journey and my love for cooking has inspired me to promote awareness about digestive health and provide people with delicious nutritious recipes that are not just gut friendly but actually gut healing. This was how my 'Heal Your Gut' cookbook series was born.

My mission is to make a difference by empowering you to improve your health and to help you on your journey to better health, whether you are suffering from serious ailments or you are on top of your health and just searching for some healthy recipes.

To learn more about my journey and how I overcame my digestive ailments, click on the image below or simply visit www.andreparker.co/healyourgut.

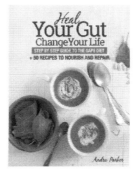

# Introduction

Welcome to the *GAPS Diet, One Pot Delights* Cookbook. I have decided to develop this book as a way to make cooking on the GAPS diet easier, healthier and more delicious. One-pot cooking is a great way to pack nutrient dense foods into your diet. In this book, I share recipes that are made using a slow cooker, sauté pans, stockpots, casserole dishes, roasting pans and even some "one bowl" condiments and desserts.

The recipes in this cookbook are specifically tailored for the GAPS diet – the Gut and Psychology Syndrome Diet. This diet was born when Dr Natasha Campbell-McBride was trying to find a way to help her son who had been diagnosed with autism. She discovered that there was a link between gut health and autism – a gut-brain connection. Dr Campbell-McBride also points to scientific data that links schizophrenia, ADHD, dyslexia, dyspraxia, asthma, allergies and eczema with gut health. She identified the key to dealing with these diseases was to heal the gut by addressing leaky gut, gut flora imbalance and nutrient deficiencies. The first step to healing our gut is to make more of our food from scratch and to include more nutrient dense gut supporting foods in our diet. This is the basis of each recipe included in this cookbook.

At this point, I would like to highlight the importance of using grass-fed and organic meats, as well as organic produce. As many of you may know, when following a dietary protocol such as GAPS, quality matters. We want to make sure that the foods we put into our body are of the highest quality to promote a healthy gut. Opt for grass-fed and organic meats whenever possible and choose organic produce to avoid exposure to pesticides or hormones. You will also find recipes for homemade bone stocks. I cannot emphasize the importance of making your own stocks enough. Some store-bought stocks are loaded with sodium and additives that we just don't want to be putting into our body. The base recipes you will find in the book are great for using as a base for many of the recipes throughout the book.

Although the focus of this book is on gut healing recipes that comply with the specific diet of GAPS, these recipes are delicious and nutritious enough for the whole family to enjoy.

Each GAPS recipe has a number next to it to indicate which stage of the diet it is suitable for.

For example:

- GAPS Stage 3+ implies that the recipe is suitable for GAPS Stage 3 and <u>onwards</u>

Please bear in mind that the ingredients and/or the method of cooking can dictate why a certain recipe is only appropriate from a certain stage. For example, cooking food by way of roasting is only recommended from stage 4 so, whilst the ingredients may comply with stage 2, the fact that they are roasted means that the recipe will be labelled as only suitable from stage 4.

Please note that each person tolerates food differently and you will be the best judge of whether or not a particular recipe is suitable for your body for the stage that it is labelled for. If you know your body reacts badly to a certain food, it's best to leave it out of the recipe, even if it technically complies with the stage you are on.

Also, please bear in mind that, if you are aware of histamine intolerance, you may wish to reduce the cooking time, especially for the stockpot recipes. For the stock recipes, it is recommended that the bones are still cooked for the length of time specified in the recipes to ensure all of the healing goodness is obtained from them, but you could consider adding the other ingredients for the last 25-30 minutes only.

The purpose of this cookbook is to share recipes with you that heal your gut but require minimal effort so that you can put nourishing and delicious meals on your dinner table each night! This book has been formulated to try to help make this easier for you. I hope that you enjoy making these dishes and that you find that they become your go-to recipes for a healthier, gut-friendly diet.

# The Different One Pot Cooking Methods & Their Benefits

**Slow Cooker:** Generally, the easiest and most time-saving method to cook one pot meals is using a slow cooker. A slow cooker is a great way to pack in a healthy dose of nutrition and make a delicious meal with minimal effort at your end.

**Vegan Slow Cooker:** These recipes are very similar to the ones found in the slow cooker section but do not contain any animal products. This is great for anyone who cannot tolerate any dairy, including ghee, or those who want to consume more plant-based recipes.

**Skillet & Sauté Pan:** These recipes are designed for the full GAPS diet as sautéing meats and vegetables in a skillet should only be introduced in the later stages of the GAPS diet. These recipes will still save you time as they only require one pan, which means less clean-up time at your end!

**Stockpot:** This is another easy way to make soups, stews and stocks. This method won't take as long as the slow cooker method so it can be very useful when you have not planned ahead or just need to throw something together unexpectedly. Making stock using a stockpot is a good way to start if you are aware of histamine intolerances – short cooked stocks are recommended for the introductory stages, if this is the case.

**Casserole Dish:** Casseroles are generally introduced during Stage 2 of the GAPS diet. You will find lots of delicious casseroles in this section where you can simply mix the ingredients, throw the dish in the oven and then enjoy the results.

**Roasting Pan:** These recipes are excellent for making meat roasts as well as roasted vegetables and you can still make an entire meal with just one pan!

**One Bowl Condiments:** A large part of the GAPS diet involves making most of your food from scratch at home. For exactly this reason, I have added a one pot condiments section to the book. You can make your own dressings and other condiments using just one jar or bowl and then enjoy them with a variety of different GAPS approved foods.

**One Bowl Desserts:** Although the GAPS diet is quite restrictive, you don't have to give up desserts completely! You will find GAPS approved desserts in this one bowl dessert section.

# The Gut and Psychology Syndrome (GAPS) Diet

If you have started reading this book, the chances are that you are probably already familiar with the GAPS diet. However, to ensure everyone is on the same page, I want to share a general breakdown of how the diet works exactly.

Firstly, I would like to stress that the best resource for determining which foods you should be introducing at each stage of the GAPS diet is Dr. Natasha Campbell's Gut and Psychology Syndrome (GAPS) book. This book will help guide you through the process so that you know exactly when it's appropriate for you to introduce certain foods. Keep in mind that each person will be different and you may have to stay at one stage longer than another. This will be where listening to your body is important.

I would like to take this opportunity to express my deepest thanks to the wonderful Dr. Natasha Campbell who developed the GAPS diet and who has helped thousands of people overcome their health issues, including me.

The GAPS diet contains six different stages, which comprise the GAPS introduction diet. Once each stage of the diet has been successfully completed, you move onto the next stage. Once you have completed stage six, you move onto the full GAPS diet. Each stage of the diet prepares you for the next stage and, as you complete each stage, you will be able to gradually include more foods.

The introduction portion of the diet is fairly restrictive when it comes to the foods that you can eat. The purpose of this is to only include foods that will help to nourish your gut and restore health. You will be removing any foods that cause irritation to the gut and focusing on foods that allow the gut to start repairing itself. You can decide to move through the diet as you see fit and according to how your body responds. You do not have to stay at one stage for any particular length of time and you may wish to stay at each stage for different lengths of time, depending on your symptoms. The key here is to just stay the course and only consume the foods that are permitted in that stage. Make sure that your symptoms are improving before moving to the next stage. Dr Campbell provides more guidance on this in her book referenced above.

Once you have completed the introduction portion of the GAPS diet, you can then move onto the full GAPS diet, which is a more sustainable approach to the GAPS way of eating. The average person typically follows the full GAPS diet for about 2 years but this time period will vary from person to person.

I have included recipes for all of the different stages of the GAPS diet so, no matter where you are with the diet, there will be something for you.

# BASE RECIPES

# Chicken Stock (GAPS Stage 1+)

**Serves:** 10
**Prep Time:** 10 minutes
**Cook Time:** 2.5 - 3.5 hours

## Ingredients:

2 lbs. of chicken pieces (legs, wings, necks)
2 quarts of filtered water
2 carrots, chopped
6 cloves of garlic, chopped
2 sprigs of fresh rosemary
5 sprigs of fresh thyme
5 sprigs of fresh parsley
1 bay leaf
1 tsp. sea salt

## Directions:

1. Simply add all of the ingredients to a large stockpot and bring to a boil. Simmer for about 3 hours.

2. Remove the chicken, keeping the meat for other recipes, if desired, and strain the stock before using.

3. Freeze any leftover stock to have on hand when you need homemade stock and are short on time.

# Beef Stock (GAPS Stage 1+)

**Serves:**      10
**Prep Time:**  10 minutes
**Cook Time:**  3 hours 20 minutes

## Ingredients:

2 lbs. beef soup bones
2 quarts of filtered water
2 carrots, chopped
6 cloves of garlic, chopped
2 sprigs of fresh rosemary
5 sprigs of fresh thyme
5 sprigs of fresh parsley
1 bay leaf
1 tsp. sea salt
1 Tbsp. olive oil

## Directions:

1. Start by heating a large stockpot over medium heat with the olive oil. Add the beef soup bones and sauté until the bones are browned. This will take about 20 minutes. Be sure to flip them periodically.

2. Add the water and remaining ingredients and bring to a boil. Simmer for about 3 hours.

3. Remove the bones and strain the stock before using.

4. Freeze any leftover stock to have on hand when you need homemade stock and are short on time.

# Fish Stock (GAPS Stage 1+)

**Serves:** 10
**Prep Time:** 10 minutes
**Cook Time:** 1 - 1.5 hours

## Ingredients:

2 lbs. of fish fins, bones and head
2 quarts of filtered water
2 carrots, chopped
½ bulb of fennel, chopped
3 cloves of garlic, chopped
2 sprigs of fresh thyme
2 sprigs of fresh parsley
1 bay leaf
1 tsp. sea salt
1 Tbsp. black peppercorns

## Directions:

1. Simply add all of the ingredients to a large stockpot and bring to a boil. Simmer for about an hour to an hour and a half.

2. Remove the fish fins, bones and head and strain the stock before using.

3. Freeze any leftover stock to have on hand when you need homemade stock and are short on time.

# Vegetable Stock (Full GAPS)

**Serves:**     10
**Prep Time:**  10 minutes
**Cook Time:**  30-35 minutes

## Ingredients:

1 onion, chopped
1 carrot, chopped
2 stalks of celery, chopped
6 cloves of garlic, chopped
2 sprigs of fresh rosemary
5 sprigs of fresh thyme
5 sprigs of fresh parsley
1 bay leaf
2 quarts of filtered water
1 tsp. sea salt
1 Tbsp. olive oil

## Directions:

1. Start by adding the olive oil to a large stock pot with the onion, garlic, carrot and celery, and cook for 5 minutes.

2. Add in the remaining ingredients and simmer for 25-30 minutes.

3. Strain the stock before using.

4. Freeze any leftover stock to have on hand when you need homemade stock and are short on time.

**Note:** Since this stock is not bone stock, it is not really suitable for the healing, introductory stages of the GAPS diet and it has therefore been labelled Full GAPS.

# SLOW COOKER RECIPES

# Gut-Soothing Vegetable Stew (GAPS Stage 1+)

**Serves:** 4
**Prep Time:** 10 minutes
**Cook Time:** 4 hours

## Ingredients:

6 cups of bone stock (homemade)
2 zucchinis, quartered
1 cup of carrots, chopped
1 garlic clove, chopped
1 yellow onion, chopped
1 tsp. fresh thyme
¼ tsp. ground peppercorn

## Directions:

1. Start by adding all of the ingredients minus the bone stock and ground peppercorn to the base of a crockpot.

2. Cover with the bone stock and season with the ground peppercorn.

3. Cook on low for 4 hours.

4. Remove the thyme and serve.

**Note:** It is recommended to remove any herbs used for flavoring before serving at this stage. Herbs are best introduced at stage 3 as they are high in fiber.

# Crock Pot Bone Stock (GAPS Stage 1+)

**Serves:**      8
**Prep Time:**   10 minutes
**Cook Time:**   8 hours

## Ingredients:

3 lbs. of beef bones
2 Tbsp. raw apple cider vinegar
Filtered water to cover
1 onion, chopped
1 bay leaf
Herbs of choice (thyme, parsley, rosemary) tied in a bouquet garni

## Directions:

1. Start by placing the beef bones in the base of a crockpot with the chopped onion and herbs.

2. Top with the filtered water and apple cider vinegar.

3. Cook on low for at least 8 hours.

4. Remove the bones and herbs, including the bay leaf, before serving.

5. Enjoy as it is or use it as a base for soups and stews.

**Note:** It is recommended to remove any herbs used for flavoring before serving at this stage. Herbs are best introduced at stage 3 as they are high in fiber.

# Asparagus Soup (GAPS Stage 1+)

**Serves:**      4
**Prep Time:**   15 minutes
**Cook Time:**   4-6 hours

## Ingredients:

1 bunch of asparagus trimmed and cut into 2-inch pieces
4 cups of bone stock (homemade)
1 yellow onion, chopped
1 clove of garlic, chopped
1 sprig of fresh dill
Sea salt and pepper to taste

## Directions:

1. Start by chopping the asparagus and placing them in the base of a crockpot.

2. Add the onion, garlic and bone stock. Stir.

3. Add in the dill, salt and pepper and cook on high for 4-6 hours.

4. Remove the dill from the soup.

5. Using an immersion blender, blend until smooth.

6. Enjoy!

**Note:** It is recommended to remove any herbs used for flavoring before serving at this stage. Herbs are best introduced at stage 3 as they are high in fiber.

# Turkey & Carrot Stew (GAPS Stage 2+)

**Serves:**      4
**Prep Time:**   10 minutes
**Cook Time:**   6-8 hours

## Ingredients:

1 lb. of turkey breast, cubed
2 cups of carrots, thinly sliced
6 cups of bone stock (homemade)
1 red onion, chopped
2 cloves of garlic, chopped
½ tsp. ground peppercorn
½ tsp. sea salt

## Directions:

1.  Add all the ingredients minus the bone stock, salt and pepper to the base of the crockpot.

2.  Cover with the bone stock and season with salt and pepper.

3.  Cook on low for 6-8 hours.

# Rosemary Lamb Stew (GAPS Stage 3+)

**Serves:**      4
**Prep Time:**   10 minutes
**Cook Time:**   6-8 hours

## Ingredients:

1 lb. of boneless leg of lamb chopped into 1 inch cubes
6 cups of bone stock (homemade)
1 butternut squash, peeled and cubed
2 carrots, thinly sliced
1 yellow onion, chopped
2 cloves of garlic, chopped
2 thyme sprigs
1 rosemary sprig
½ tsp. sea salt
½ tsp. black pepper

## Directions:

1.  Start by adding the lamb, carrots, butternut squash, onion and garlic to the base of the crockpot.

2.  Cover with the bone stock, thyme and rosemary.

3.  Season with salt and pepper and cook on low for 6-8 hours or until the lamb is tender.

# Classic Gut-Health Chicken Soup (GAPS Stage 3+)

**Serves:** 4
**Prep Time:** 10 minutes
**Cook Time:** 7 hours

## Ingredients:

4 boneless skinless chicken breasts
1 butternut squash, peeled and cubed
2 cups of carrots, chopped
1 medium onion, diced
2 cloves of garlic, chopped
6 cups of bone stock (homemade)
1 cup of filtered water
2 Tbsp. fresh parsley, chopped

## Directions:

1. Place the chicken breasts in the base of a crockpot with the onion, garlic, carrots and butternut squash.

2. Cover with the bone stock and water

3. Cook on low for 7 hours.

4. Remove the chicken from the crockpot and either shred the chicken using two forks or cut into cubes. Return the chicken to the crockpot along with the freshly chopped parsley and stir.

5. Enjoy and store any leftovers in the fridge or freeze for later use.

# Healing Stewed Cabbage (GAPS Stage 4+)

**Serves:** 4
**Prep Time:** 10 minutes
**Cook Time:** 4 hours

## Ingredients:

1 head of cabbage, chopped
1 small yellow onion, chopped
1 garlic clove, chopped
8 cups of bone stock (homemade)
¼ cup coconut oil
1 bay leaf
Sea salt and pepper to taste

## Directions:

1. Start by placing the cabbage in the base of your crockpot and top with the onion, garlic, coconut oil, bay leaf and bone stock.

2. Season with salt and pepper.

3. Cook on high for 4 hours.

4. Remove the bay leaf before serving.

# Slow Cooker Butternut Squash Soup (GAPS Stage 6+)

**Serves:** 4
**Prep Time:** 10 minutes
**Cook Time:** 4-6 hours

## Ingredients:

2 cups of butternut squash, cubed
6 cups of bone stock (homemade)
1 garlic clove, chopped
1 yellow onion, chopped
1 cup of homemade coconut milk
1 rosemary sprig
Sea salt and pepper to taste
Cracked red pepper for garnish (optional)

## Directions:

1. Place the butternut squash, onion and garlic in the base of the crockpot.

2. Top with the bone stock and rosemary, and season with salt and pepper.

3. Cook on high for 4-6 hours. During the last hour of cook time, add in the full-fat coconut milk and stir.

4. Remove the rosemary sprig before serving.

5. Serve with cracked red pepper, if desired.

**Quick Tip:** This recipe is suitable for GAPS Stage 2+ if the coconut milk and cracked red pepper is omitted and the rosemary sprig is removed before serving.

# Creamy Fennel Soup (Full GAPS)

**Serves:**      4
**Prep Time:**   15 minutes
**Cook Time:**   4-6 hours

## Ingredients:

1 fennel bulb
1 white onion
4 cups of bone stock (homemade)
1 cup of homemade coconut milk
1 tsp. cumin
Sea salt and pepper to taste
1 Tbsp. fresh dill for serving (optional)

## Directions:

1.  Start by chopping the fennel bulb and placing it in the base of a crockpot.

2.  Cover with the onion and bone stock, and add the seasoning. Stir.

3.  Cook on high for 4-6 hours. During the last hour of cooking time, add in the full-fat coconut milk and stir.

4.  Using an immersion blender, blend until smooth and serve with fresh dill, if desired.

# Coconut Mushroom Soup (Full GAPS)

**Serves:** 4
**Prep Time:** 15 minutes
**Cook Time:** 4-6 hours

## Ingredients:

½ cup of mushrooms, sliced
4 cups of bone stock (homemade)
¼ cup homemade coconut milk
1 yellow onion, chopped
1 clove of garlic, chopped
¼ tsp. ground nutmeg
Sea salt and pepper to taste

## Directions:

1. Start by chopping the mushrooms and placing them in the base of a crockpot.

2. Cover with the onion, garlic and bone stock, and add the seasoning. Stir.

3. Cook on high for 4-6 hours. During the last hour of cook time, add in the full-fat coconut milk and stir.

4. Using an immersion blender blend until smooth.

# VEGAN SLOW COOKER

# Celery Dill Soup (Full GAPS)

**Serves:** 4
**Prep Time:** 15 minutes
**Cook Time:** 4-6 hours

## Ingredients:

1 cup of homemade vegetable stock
4 celery stalks, chopped
1 bulb of fennel, chopped
2 garlic cloves, chopped
2 Tbsp. fresh dill
Sea salt and pepper to taste

## Directions:

1. Simply add all ingredients to the base of a crockpot and cook on high for 4-6 hours.

2. Using an immersion blender, blend the soup until smooth.

3. Enjoy.

**Note:** This recipe has been labelled Full GAPS due to the high fiber content of celery. You may be able to introduce cooked celery from Stage 3 without any adverse effects but my recommendation would be to wait until Full GAPS.

# Vegan Creamy Carrot Soup (Full GAPS)

**Serves:**     4
**Prep Time:**   15 minutes
**Cook Time:** 6 hours

## Ingredients:

1 lb. of carrots, chopped
1 yellow onion, chopped
2 cloves of garlic, chopped
2 cups of homemade vegetable stock
½ tsp. freshly grated ginger
¼ tsp. ground nutmeg
Sea salt and pepper to taste

## Directions:

1.  Start by adding the carrots, onion and garlic to the base of a slow cooker.

2.  Add the vegetable stock and seasoning.

3.  Cook on low for 6 hours.

4.  Using an immersion blender, blend until smooth.

5.  Enjoy.

# Cream of Pumpkin Soup (Full GAPS)

**Serves:**     4
**Prep Time:**  15 minutes
**Cook Time:**  6-8 hours

## Ingredients:

4 cups of homemade vegetable stock
2 cups of fresh pumpkin diced
1 large carrot, chopped
1 onion, chopped
2 cloves of garlic, chopped
1 winter squash, cubed
1 cup of homemade coconut milk
Sea salt and pepper to taste

## Directions:

1. Start by adding all of the ingredients to a slow cooker minus the coconut milk and cook on low for 6-8 hours.

2. During the last hour of cooking time, add the coconut milk and stir.

3. Using an immersion blender, blend the soup until smooth.

4. Season with salt and pepper and enjoy.

# Garlic & Kale Soup (Full GAPS)

**Serves:**     4
**Prep Time:**   15 minutes
**Cook Time:**  5-6 hours

## Ingredients:

4 cups of homemade vegetable stock
4 cups of fresh kale, chopped
3 cloves of garlic, chopped
1 red onion, chopped
1 cup of dry white navy beans, rinsed and soaked (for 8 hours in the fridge)
1 tsp. coriander
1 tsp. fresh dill
Sea salt and pepper to taste

## Directions:

1. Start by adding all of the ingredients to a slow cooker and cook on high for 5-6 hours or until the beans are tender.

2. Using an immersion blender, blend the soup until smooth.

3. Enjoy.

# Gut-Healing Vegetable Soup (Full GAPS)

**Serves:** 4
**Prep Time:** 10 minutes
**Cook Time:** 5-6 hours

## Ingredients:

6 cups of homemade vegetable stock
1 cup of fresh kale, chopped
1 bulb of fennel, chopped
2 cloves of garlic, chopped
1 large carrot, chopped
1 winter squash, cubed
1 cup of dry white navy beans, rinsed and soaked (for 8 hours in the fridge)
1 tsp. coriander
Sea salt and pepper to taste

## Directions:

1. Start by adding all of the ingredients to a slow cooker and cook on high for 5-6 hours or until the beans are tender.

2. Stir and enjoy.

# SKILLET & SAUTE PAN

# Zucchini & Carrot Noodles with Lime (GAPS Stage 4+)

**Serves:** 2
**Prep Time:** 10 minutes
**Cook Time:** 5 minutes

## Ingredients:

4 large carrots, washed
2 large zucchinis
2 cloves of garlic, chopped
2 Tbsp. freshly squeezed lime juice
1 Tbsp. cold pressed olive oil
1 tsp. oregano
1 tsp. basil
Sea salt and pepper to taste
Cold pressed olive oil for cooking

## Directions:

1. Start by heating a large skillet over medium heat with the olive oil for cooking.

2. Spiralize the zucchinis and carrots using a spiralizer or mandolin.

3. Add the zucchinis, carrots and garlic to the skillet and cook for about 5 minutes or until tender.

4. Remove from heat and drizzle with the lime juice and olive oil.

5. Season with oregano, basil, salt and pepper.

# "Creamed" Spinach (Full GAPS)

**Serves:** 3
**Prep Time:** 10 minutes
**Cook Time:** 8-11 minutes

## Ingredients:

6 cups of fresh spinach
2 cloves of garlic, chopped
1 Tbsp. freshly squeezed lemon juice
1 Tbsp. ghee
¼ cup homemade coconut milk
Sea salt and pepper to taste

## Directions:

1. Start by heating a large skillet over low heat with the ghee. Add the fresh spinach and garlic and sauté for 3-4 minutes or until the spinach begins to wilt.

2. Add the remaining ingredients and allow the coconut milk to cook down for about 5-7 minutes.

3. Season with salt and pepper and enjoy with a side of cooked chicken or lamb.

**Quick Tip:** This recipe is suitable for GAPS Stage 3+ if the coconut milk is omitted.

# Ground Taco Meat (Full GAPS)

**Serves:**      4
**Prep Time:**   10 minutes
**Cook Time:**   15 minutes

## Ingredients:

1 lb. of organic ground turkey
2 cloves of garlic, chopped
1 red onion, chopped
1 tsp. coriander
1 Tbsp. fresh parsley
Coconut oil for cooking
Sea salt and pepper to taste

## Directions:

1. Start by heating a large skillet over medium heat with the coconut oil. Add the ground turkey and cook until thoroughly cooked through.

2. Add the remaining ingredients and cook for another 5 minutes.

3. Serve with large lettuce leaves for a traditional style "taco" with sliced tomatoes and avocado.

# Grass Fed Beef Burgers (Full GAPS)

**Serves:**    4
**Prep Time:**    15 minutes
**Cook Time:**    10 minutes

## Ingredients:

1 lb. of grass-fed organic beef
2 cloves of garlic, chopped
1 red onion, chopped
1 tsp. coriander
1 tsp. cumin
½ tsp. ground turmeric
1 Tbsp. fresh parsley
Coconut oil for cooking
Sea salt and pepper to taste

## Directions:

1. Start by heating a large skillet over medium heat with the coconut oil.

2. Add the beef with the remaining ingredients to a large mixing bowl and stir to combine.

3. Form the burger mixture into 4 patties and cook on the skillet for about 5 minutes each side or until cooked to your liking.

4. Serve with large lettuce leaves instead of a bun and add sliced avocado, if desired.

# Turkey Skillet Meatballs (Full GAPS)

**Serves:** 8
**Prep Time:** 15 minutes
**Cook Time:** 14 minutes

## Ingredients:

1 lb. of organic ground turkey
1 organic pasture-raised egg
2 cloves of garlic, chopped
1 Tbsp. fresh parsley
Coconut oil for cooking
Sea salt and pepper to taste

## Directions:

1. Start by heating a large skillet over medium heat with the coconut oil.

2. Add the ground turkey and egg to a mixing bowl and stir to combine.

3. Add the chopped garlic, fresh parsley, salt and pepper. Stir again and then form into small meatballs.

4. Add to the skillet and cook for about 7 minutes on each side or until the outside of the meatballs are browned and cooked through.

5. Serve with cooked squash or spiralized zucchini, if desired.

# Vegetable & Chicken Kabobs (Full GAPS)

**Serves:**      3
**Prep Time:**   15 minutes
**Cook Time:**   20 minutes

## Ingredients:

3 chicken breasts, cubed
1 yellow bell pepper, chopped
6 garlic cloves, whole
1 red onion, quartered
1 Tbsp. fresh rosemary
2 Tbsp. cold pressed virgin olive oil
Sea salt and pepper to taste
Kabob sticks

## Directions:

1. Start by heating a large skillet over medium heat with the olive oil.

2. Add the chicken to the pan first and cook until thoroughly cooked through.

3. Add the vegetables, rosemary, salt and pepper. Cook for another 5 minutes.

4. Add the cubed chicken and vegetables to the kabob sticks in any order you desire and enjoy.

# Garlic & Thyme Lamb Chops (Full GAPS)

**Serves:** 4
**Prep Time:** 35 minutes
**Cook Time:** 6-10 minutes

## Ingredients:

8 organic grass-fed lamb chops
3 garlic cloves, whole
1 Tbsp. fresh thyme
2 Tbsp. virgin cold pressed olive oil
Sea salt and pepper to taste

## Directions:

1. Start by seasoning the lamb chops with the fresh thyme and 1 tablespoon of the olive oil. Place in the refrigerator for 30 minutes to marinate.

2. When ready to cook, preheat a large skillet over medium heat with the other 1 tablespoon of olive oil and cook the lamb chops with the whole garlic cloves for about 3-5 minutes on each side or until cooked to your liking.

3. Enjoy with steamed broccoli or asparagus.

# Mushroom Cabbage Stir Fry (Full GAPS)

**Serves:** 4
**Prep Time:** 10 minutes
**Cook Time:** 12-15 minutes

## Ingredients:

1 head of cabbage, chopped
1 cup of button mushrooms, chopped
1 whole organic rotisserie chicken, shredded
2 cloves of garlic, chopped
1 Tbsp. fresh thyme
2 Tbsp. virgin cold pressed olive oil
Sea salt and pepper to taste

## Directions:

1. Start by heating a large skillet over medium heat with the olive oil. Add the cabbage and mushrooms and sauté for about 7-10 minutes or until the cabbage begins to wilt.

2. Add the remaining ingredients and stir. Cook for another 5 minutes.

3. Season with salt and pepper and enjoy.

# Bolognese Sauce (Full GAPS)

**Serves:** 8
**Prep Time:** 10 minutes
**Cook Time:** 8-15 minutes

## Ingredients:

1 lb. of grass-fed ground beef
1 Tbsp. coconut oil
1 onion, chopped
3 cloves of garlic, chopped
5 tomatoes, diced
1 tsp. oregano
1 tsp. basil
Sea salt and pepper to taste

## Directions:

1. Start by heating a large skillet over medium heat with the coconut oil.

2. Add the ground beef and brown for 3-5 minutes.

3. Add in the remaining ingredients and cook for another 5-10 minutes or until the beef is cooked through and the vegetables are tender.

4. Serve with a side of fresh vegetables or spiralized zucchini.

**Quick Tip:** This recipe is suitable for GAPS Stage 4+ if cooked in a stockpot with a little bit of homemade stock instead.

# STOCKPOT

# Ratatouille (GAPS Stage 4+)

**Serves:** 6
**Prep time:** 15 minutes
**Cook time:** 30 minutes

## Ingredients:

- 3 Tbsp. coconut oil
- 1 large onion, chopped
- 1 tsp. sea salt
- 4 cloves garlic, chopped
- 2 tsp. oregano
- 1 bell pepper, chopped
- 1 small eggplant, cut into bit-sized cubes
- 2 zucchinis, chopped
- 4 cups tomatoes, chopped
- 1 cup bone stock

## Directions:

1. In a large pot, heat 3 tablespoons of coconut oil over medium heat. Add the onion and salt, and sauté until translucent, about 3 minutes.

2. Add the garlic, oregano, bell pepper, eggplant and zucchinis and cook for 5 minutes, stirring frequently.

3. Add the chopped tomatoes and bone stock, bring to a boil then reduce heat to low and simmer, covered, for 20-30 minutes or until vegetables are cooked through.

4. Add salt and pepper to taste.

# Turmeric Ginger Chicken Soup (GAPS Stage 3+)

**Serves**       4
**Prep time:**   10 minutes
**Cook time:**   45 minutes

## Ingredients:

2 Tbsp. coconut oil
1 onion, chopped
½ tsp. sea salt
3 cloves garlic, chopped
1 Tbsp. fresh grated ginger
1 Tbsp. fresh grated turmeric
2 cups sliced mushrooms
2 lb. chicken thighs
6 cups bone stock

## Directions:

1. In a large pot, heat the coconut oil over medium heat. Add the onion and salt and cook until translucent, about 3 minutes.

2. Add the garlic, ginger, turmeric and mushrooms and cook for 1 minute, stirring frequently.

3. Add the chicken thighs and bone stock. Bring to a boil then reduce heat to low and simmer for 45 minutes or until the chicken is cooked through.

4. Remove the chicken from the pot and shred using two forks. Return to the pot and add salt and pepper to taste.

# Simple Beef Chili (Full GAPS)

**Serves:** 4-6
**Prep time:** 10 minutes
**Cook time:** 1-1.5 hours

## Ingredients:

1 Tbsp. coconut oil

2 lbs. grass-fed beef stew meat

2 bell peppers, chopped

2 tsp. garlic powder

2 tsp. onion powder

2 tsp. oregano

2 tsp. cumin

½ tsp. cinnamon

2 tsp. sea salt

4 cups chopped tomatoes

2 cups bone stock

## Directions:

1. In a large pot, heat the coconut oil over medium-high heat.

2. Add the beef stew meat and cook to brown on all sides.

3. Use a slotted spoon to remove from the pot onto a plate.

4. Add the bell peppers, garlic powder, onion powder, oregano, cumin, cinnamon and salt.

5. Cook until fragrant, about 1 minute.

6. Return the meat to the pot along with the chopped tomatoes and bone stock.

7. Reduce heat to simmer and cook, covered, until beef is cooked through, about 1-1.5 hours.

8. Season with salt and pepper to taste.

**Quick Tip:** This recipe is suitable for GAPS Stage 4+ if cooked in a stockpot with a little bit of homemade stock instead and the cinnamon, onion powder and garlic powder are omitted and replaced with diced onion and garlic.

# Pumpkin Chicken Curry (Full GAPS)

**Serves:**      4
**Prep time:**   10 minutes
**Cook time:**  20 minutes

## Ingredients:

2 Tbsp. coconut oil
1 onion, chopped
1 tsp. salt
1 Tbsp. curry powder
1 lb. pumpkin or other squash, peeled and chopped into small cubes
1 lb. chicken thighs, cut into bite-sized pieces
2 ½ cups homemade coconut milk
1 cup bone stock
1 lime, cut into wedges

## Directions:

1. In a large pot, heat the coconut oil over medium heat. Add the onion and salt and cook until translucent, about 3 minutes.

2. Add the curry powder and pumpkin and cook for 1 minute, stirring frequently.

3. Add in the chicken, coconut milk and bone stock.

4. Bring to a boil then reduce heat to low and simmer for 15 minutes or until the chicken and pumpkin are cooked through.

5. Season with salt and pepper to taste.

6. Serve with a squeeze of lime.

# CASSEROLE DISH

# Smoky Baked Eggs and Butternut Squash (GAPS Stage 4+)

**Serves:** 4
**Prep time:** 10 minutes
**Cook time:** 35 minutes

## Ingredients:

1.5 lb. butternut squash, peeled, seeds removed and halved
2 Tbsp. olive oil
2 tsp. smoked paprika
1 tsp. ground turmeric
½ tsp. sea salt
4 organic pasture-raised eggs

## Directions:

1. Preheat the oven to 425°F.

2. In a 9x13 casserole dish, add the butternut squash, olive oil, smoked paprika, turmeric and salt and toss to coat.

3. Bake for 25 minutes or until fork tender. Remove from the oven and create four small holes in the butternut squash.

4. Crack an egg into each hole and bake for 10 more minutes or until the eggs are set.

# Riced Cauliflower and Meatballs (GAPS Stage 4+)

**Serves:** 3-4
**Prep time:** 15 minutes
**Cook time:** 20 minutes

## Ingredients:

1 head cauliflower, chopped finely
4 cups chopped tomatoes
2 Tbsp. cold pressed olive oil
4 cloves garlic, minced
1 tsp. sea salt

## For the meatballs:

1 lb. grass-fed ground beef
1 organic pasture-raised egg
¼ cup almond flour (preferably homemade by grinding almonds in a food processor)
1 Tbsp. dried oregano
½ tsp. sea salt

## Directions:

1. Preheat the oven to 400°F.

2. In a 9x13 casserole dish, mix together the cauliflower, chopped tomatoes, olive oil, garlic and salt.

3. For the meatballs, combine all ingredients in a bowl and use your hands to mix everything together. Roll into meatballs.

4. Nestle the meatballs in the cauliflower. Bake for 15-20 minutes or until cooked through.

# Butternut Casserole (GAPS Stage 6+)

**Serves:** 4
**Prep Time:** 15 minutes
**Cook Time:** 25-30 minutes

## Ingredients:

4 cups of butternut squash, peeled and cubed
½ cup of chopped carrots
4 Tbsp. melted coconut oil
4 Tbsp. homemade coconut milk
1 tsp. ground cinnamon
Sea salt and pepper to taste

## Directions:

1. Start by preheating the oven to 350°F and greasing a casserole dish.

2. Add the butternut squash and carrots to the casserole dish with the remaining ingredients and gently stir to combine.

3. Place in the oven and cook for 25-30 minutes or until the butternut squash and carrots are tender.

4. Sprinkle with extra ground cinnamon, if desired.

# Lemon Chicken and Broccoli (Full GAPS)

**Serves:** 4
**Prep time:** 10 minutes
**Cook time:** 25 minutes

## Ingredients:

4 chicken breasts, cut into cubes
1 head broccoli, cut into small florets
2 cups sliced mushrooms
1 tsp. sea salt
1 Tbsp. olive oil
2 lemons, sliced into thin rounds
½ cup homemade coconut milk
1 cup bone stock

## Directions:

1. Preheat oven to 400°F. In a 9x13 casserole dish, add the chicken, broccoli, mushrooms, salt and olive oil and toss to coat.

2. Arrange the lemon slices on top.

3. Add the coconut milk and bone stock, and bake for 25 minutes or until the chicken is cooked through.

# Italian Egg Bake (GAPS Stage 6+)

**Serves:**       4
**Prep time:**    15 minutes
**Cook time:**    40 minutes

## Ingredients:

10 organic pasture-raised eggs
¼ cup homemade coconut milk
1 Tbsp. oregano
2 tsp. sea salt
5 cloves garlic, minced
1 large tomato, chopped
2 small zucchinis, sliced
1 cup fresh basil, chopped or 2 Tbsp. dried basil

## Directions:

1.  Preheat the oven to 375°F. In a 9x13 casserole dish, whisk together the eggs, coconut milk, oregano and salt.

2.  Mix in the garlic, tomato and zucchinis. Top with fresh or dried basil.

3.  Bake for 40 minutes or until the eggs are set in the center.

**Quick Tip:** This recipe may be suitable for Stage 4 if the coconut milk is omitted.

# ROASTING PAN

# Lemon Garlic Roasted Chicken (GAPS Stage 4+)

**Serves:** 8
**Prep Time:** 20 minutes
**Cook Time:** 1 ½ hours

## Ingredients:

1.5 lb. organic grass-fed roasting chicken
1 lemon, sliced
2 Tbsp. extra virgin olive oil
1 head of garlic, cut in half
1 Tbsp. fresh thyme
3 rosemary sprigs
Sea salt and pepper to taste

## Directions:

1. Start by preheating the oven to 450°F and greasing a roasting pan.

2. Remove the chicken giblets and rinse the chicken under cool water. Pat dry and add to the roasting pan.

3. Season with salt, pepper and fresh thyme.

4. Fill the cavity of the chicken with the lemon, garlic and rosemary sprigs.

5. Brush the outside of the chicken with the olive oil.

6. Tie the legs of the chicken using kitchen string and then tuck the wings under.

7. Place in the oven and bake for an hour and a half or until the juices start to run clear and the chicken is cooked through.

8. Allow the chicken to sit out for about 10-15 minutes before slicing.

# Garlic Beef Roast (GAPS Stage 4+)

**Serves:**      8
**Prep Time:**   20 minutes
**Cook Time:**   60 minutes

## Ingredients:

3 lb. organic grass-fed beef roast
2 large carrots
4 cloves of garlic
Sea salt and pepper to taste

## Directions:

1. Start by preheating the oven to 375°F and greasing a roasting pan.

2. Place the roast into the roasting pan and season with salt and pepper.

3. Add the carrots and garlic to the bottom of the roasting pan.

4. Roast for an hour or 20 minutes per pound if you are using a larger or smaller roast. You can increase the cooking time according to how well done you want your roast.

5. Allow the roast to sit out for about 10-15 minutes before slicing.

# Roasted Thyme Lamb Chops (GAPS Stage 4+)

**Serves:** 4
**Prep Time:** 15 minutes
**Cook Time:** 10-20 minutes

## Ingredients:

2 racks of lamb
1 Tbsp. fresh thyme
1 clove of garlic, chopped
2 Tbsp. extra virgin olive oil
Sea salt and pepper to taste

## Directions:

1. Start by preheating the oven to 400°F and greasing a roasting pan.

2. Place the lamb chops into the roasting pan and season with the olive oil, thyme, garlic, salt and pepper.

3. Roast for 10-20 minutes or until cooked to your liking.

4. Enjoy with a side of roasted or steamed vegetables.

# Roasted Zucchini (GAPS Stage 4+)

**Serves:**      4
**Prep Time:**   10 minutes
**Cook Time:**   30-35 minutes

## Ingredients:

2 large zucchinis, sliced
2 Tbsp. coconut oil, melted
1 garlic clove, chopped
1 tsp. oregano
1 tsp. Celtic sea salt

## Directions:

1. Start by preheating the oven to 350°F and greasing a roasting pan.

2. Add the sliced zucchinis to the roasting pan, drizzle with coconut oil and season with the garlic, oregano and salt.

3. Bake for 30-35 minutes.

# Roasted Pumpkin (GAPS Stage 4+)

**Serves:**     4
**Prep Time:**  15 minutes
**Cook Time:**  30-35 minutes

## Ingredients:

1 large pumpkin, peeled, seeded and cut into cubes
2 Tbsp. coconut oil, melted
1 garlic clove, chopped
1 tsp. fresh rosemary
1 tsp. fresh thyme
1 tsp. Celtic sea salt

## Directions:

1.  Start by preheating the oven to 450°F and greasing a roasting pan.

2.  Add the cubed pumpkin to the roasting pan, drizzle with the coconut oil and season with the garlic, rosemary, thyme and salt.

3.  Roast for 30-35 minutes, tossing halfway through.

# "ONE BOWL" CONDIMENTS

# Lemon Dressing & Marinade (GAPS Stage 4+)

**Serves:** 8
**Prep Time:** 5 minutes
**Cook Time:** 0 minutes

## Ingredients:

- 1 cup of extra virgin olive oil
- ¼ cup lemon juice, freshly squeezed
- 1 garlic clove, chopped
- 1 Tbsp. fresh parsley, chopped
- 1 tsp. Celtic sea salt

## Directions:

1. Simply place all ingredients into a glass bowl or jar and, using an immersion blender, blend until smooth.

2. Store in the refrigerator until ready to use.

# Homemade Ketchup (GAPS Stage 6+)

**Serves:**     10
**Prep Time:**  5 minutes
**Cook Time:**  0 minutes

## Ingredients:

1 ½ cups pure tomato puree
¼ cup raw honey
2 Tbsp. raw apple cider vinegar
1 Tbsp. ghee
1 tsp. ground cinnamon
1 tsp. sea salt

## Directions:

1. Add all the ingredients to a large bowl and whisk to combine.

2. Transfer to a mason style glass jar and store in the refrigerator.

# Homemade Mayonnaise (Full GAPS)

**Serves:** 10
**Prep Time:** 5 minutes
**Cook Time:** 0 minutes

## Ingredients:

1 organic pasture-raised egg
1 Tbsp. raw apple cider vinegar
¾ cup extra virgin olive oil
½ tsp. pure mustard powder
1 tsp. sea salt

## Directions:

1. Start by adding the olive oil, egg and mustard powder to a large mason style jar and, using an immersion blender, blend until creamy.

2. Add in the raw apple cider vinegar and sea salt and blend again.

3. Store leftovers in the refrigerator.

# Avocado Dill Salad Dressing (Full GAPS)

**Serves:**     8
**Prep Time:**  5 minutes
**Cook Time:**  0 minutes

## Ingredients:

1 cup of extra virgin olive oil
1 avocado, pitted and peeled
2 Tbsp. homemade mayonnaise
1 Tbsp. freshly squeezed lemon juice
1 tsp. fresh dill, chopped
1 tsp. fresh parsley, chopped
1 garlic clove, chopped
1 tsp. Celtic sea salt

## Directions:

1. Simply place all ingredients into a glass bowl or jar and, using an immersion blender, blend until smooth.

2. Store in the refrigerator until ready to use.

# Ranch Dressing (Full GAPS)

**Serves:** 8
**Prep Time:** 5 minutes
**Cook Time:** 0 minutes

## Ingredients:

   1 cup of homemade mayonnaise
   ¼ cup avocado oil
   2 Tbsp. fresh parsley, chopped
   1 tsp. fresh dill, chopped
   1 Tbsp. lemon juice, freshly squeezed
   1 tsp. Celtic sea salt

## Directions:

1.  Simply place all ingredients into a glass bowl or jar and, using an immersion blender, blend until smooth.

2.  Store in the refrigerator until ready to use.

# ONE POT DESSERTS

# Apple Cinnamon Pancakes (Full GAPS)

**Serves:**      4
**Prep Time:**   10 minutes
**Cook Time:**  4 minutes

## Ingredients:

4 organic pasture-raised eggs
¼ cup full-fat homemade coconut milk
4 apples, peeled and grated
2 Tbsp. coconut oil
¼ cup shredded, unsweetened coconut
1 Tbsp. ground cinnamon
Coconut oil for cooking

## Directions:

1. Start by adding all ingredients to a large mixing bowl and whisk to combine.

2. Preheat a large skillet over medium heat with the coconut oil.

3. Pour a quarter of a cup of the batter into the pan and cook each pancake for about 2 minutes each side or until brown.

4. Sprinkle with extra ground cinnamon, if desired.

# Creamy Coconut Ice Cream (Full GAPS)

**Serves:** 6
**Prep Time:** 5 minutes + 4 hours in the freezer
**Cook Time:** 0 minutes

## Ingredients:

2 cups of unsweetened, full-fat coconut cream (refrigerated overnight)
¼ cup raw honey
1 tsp. ground cinnamon

## Directions:

1. Simply add all ingredients to a large mixing bowl and, either using a hand-help mixer or whisking by hand, whisk until creamy.

2. Transfer to a freezer safe container and freeze for 4 hours, stirring every hour until a soft serve ice cream consistency forms.

# Banana Milkshake (Full GAPS)

**Serves:**     2
**Prep Time:**  5 minutes
**Cook Time:**  0 minutes

## Ingredients:

 1 cup of homemade coconut milk
 1 very ripe banana
 1 Tbsp. raw honey
 ½ tsp. ground cinnamon

## Directions:

1.  Place all of the ingredients into a high-speed blender and blend until smooth.

2.  Enjoy.

# Coconut Bites (Full GAPS)

**Serves:** 10
**Prep Time:** 10 minutes + 1 hour in the fridge
**Cook Time:** 0 minutes

## Ingredients:

    1 cup of shredded, unsweetened coconut
    1 Tbsp. coconut oil
    2 Tbsp. raw honey
    ½ tsp. ground cinnamon
    Pinch of Celtic sea salt

## Directions:

1. Add all ingredients to a mixing bowl and stir to combine.

2. Form into small rounds and place back into the bowl, trying to evenly distribute them so that they are not all piled on top of one another. Refrigerate for 1 hour before serving.

3. Store leftovers in the fridge for a couple of days. You can also freeze these so that they keep for longer.

# Cooking Conversion Tables

| Spoon, Cups | Liquid - ml |
|---|---|
| 1/4 tsp. | 1.25ml |
| 1/2 tsp. | 2.5 ml |
| 1 tsp. | 5 ml |
| 1 Tbsp. | 15ml |
| 1/4 cup | 60ml |
| 1/3 cup | 80ml |
| 1/2 cup | 125 ml |
| 1 cup | 250 ml |

| Dry Measurements | | |
|---|---|---|
| 1 Tbsp. | 1/2 ounce | 14g |
| 1/4 cup | 2 ounce | 56.7g |
| 1/3 cup | 2.6 ounce | 75.4g |
| 1/2 cup | 4 ounces | 113.4 |
| 3/4 cup | 6 ounces | 170g |
| 1 cup | 8 ounces | 227g |
| 2 cups | 16 ounces | 454g |

| Volume Liquid | | |
|---|---|---|
| 2 Tbsp. | 1 fl. oz. | 30 ml |
| 1/4 cup | 2 fl. oz. | 60 ml |
| 1/2 cup | 4 fl. oz. | 125 ml |
| 1 cup | 8 fl. oz. | 250 ml |
| 1.5 cups | 12 fl. oz. | 375 ml |
| 2 cups/1 pint | 16 fl. oz. | 500 ml |
| 4 cups/1 quart | 32 fl. oz. | 1000 ml / 1 liter |

# YOU MAY ALSO LIKE

To view all the other delicious books by Andre Parker, visit the link below.

http://www.andreparker.co/amazon

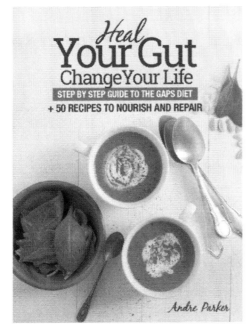

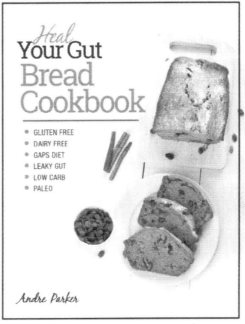

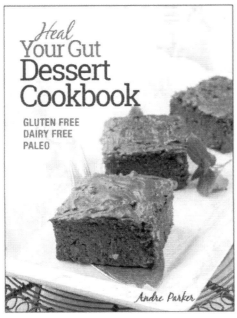

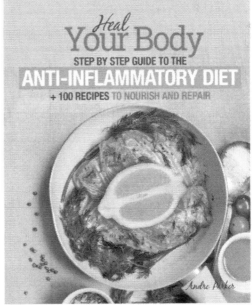

| Book Cover Design: | Karen Hue |
| Book Cover Images: | Victoria Shibut © www.123rf.com |

For more information, please contact:
ANDRE PARKER
http://www.andreparker.co
info@andreparker.co

Made in the USA
San Bernardino, CA
13 June 2018